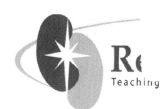

Teaching You To Master Your Health

Eating A Pre-Dialysis Kidney Diet (Stages 1 – 4) — Calories, Carbohydrates, Protein, and Fat

Book 1

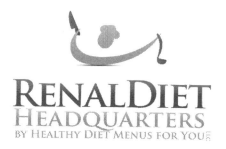

RENALDIET
HEADQUARTERS
BY HEALTHY DIET MENUS FOR YOU

PURPOSE AND INTRODUCTION

What I have found through the emails and requests of my readers is that it is difficult to find information about a pre-dialysis kidney diet that is actionable. I want you to know that is what I intend to provide in all my books. You can take these recipes from our website and information to create meals that you and your family will enjoy and they all fit a stage 2 – 5 kidney disease patient.

I wrote this book with you in mind: the person with kidney problems who does not know where to start or can't seem to get the answers that you need from other sources. This book will provide information that is applicable to a predialysis kidney disease diet.

Who am I? I am a registered dietitian in the USA who has been working with kidney patients for my entire 15 + years of experience. Find all my books on Amazon on my author page: http://www.amazon.com/Mathea-Ford/e/B008E1E7IS/

My goals are simple – to give some answers and to create an understanding of what is typical. In this series of 12 books, I will take you through the different parts of being a person with pre-dialysis kidney disease. It will not necessarily be what happens in your case, as everyone is an individual. I may simplify things in an effort to write them so that I feel you can learn the most from the information. This may mean that I don't say the exact things that your doctor would say. If you don't understand, please ask your doctor.

I want you to know, I am not a medical doctor and I am not aware of your particular condition. Information in this book is current as of publication, but may or may not have changed. This book is not meant to substitute for medical treatment for you, your friends, your caregivers, or your family members. You should not base treatment decisions solely on what is contained in this book. Develop your treatment plan with your doctors, nurses and the other medical professionals on your team. I recommend that you double-check any information with your medical team to verify if it applies to you.

In other words, I am not responsible for your medical care. I am providing this book for information and entertainment purposes, not medical diagnoses. Please consult with your doctor about any questions that you have about your particular case.

TABLE OF CONTENTS

OVERVIEW OF THE PRE-DIALYSIS KIDNEY DIET

Food is one of the few things we cannot avoid. We have to eat something in order to survive. And I suspect that at this point you might feel like food is your enemy. But making meals for yourself or your family should not be painful. This book is designed to provide you with a guide that will take you from misunderstanding and frustration to peace and harmony with your body. Improving your health as well. The food you eat should provide you with comfort and joy.

You probably have foods that you like or don't like. You possibly have foods that you used to eat but no longer eat. Or you might just eat about anything. Whether you are overweight or underweight or at a healthy weight – you need to eat something. And right now, with kidney disease, you need that food to nourish and provide the kind of healthy meal that will feed your kidneys to improve your health, not further their damage.

You will experience changes to your lifestyle and habits. I hope that you are open to changing some things, because your success on this diet will be dependent on your flexibility and openness to changes in the way you prepare and eat food. Kidney disease, like many chronic illnesses, can cause you to rethink your routine and change your eating and drinking habits. It might feel like it's hard to understand and even harder to implement, but that is why I wrote this book. To help you get a handle on what changes need to be made and how to make them.

Regardless of the stage of kidney disease you have, you need to understand the underlying causes and reasons for the way the diet is. I am sure that you are concerned about eating just the right thing to slow down the damage that is happening to your kidneys.

You are going to learn the reasons why we have the diet, what it does, where you should be focusing on and what you should learn in this book.

What Is The Purpose Of The Diet?

The reason why we have a kidney diet for "pre-dialysis" is so that we can slow down the damage that is happening to your kidneys. Your kidneys are remarkable machines, and they filter millions of gallons of waste out of your blood, but somehow they were damaged and are not working quite as efficiently. You might have found out you are in Stage 3 and wonder what that means. The damage to your kidneys is from the food you eat and your related conditions. If you have high blood pressure or diabetes, you need to get them under control immediately. Your blood pressure damages the tiny blood vessels in your kidneys that filter the blood. Diabetes damages kidneys with the excess blood sugar levels. When recommendations are made, they are made to slow or stop the progression of damage to the capillaries in your kidneys. Never fear, you don't have to understand how kidneys work to get a good diet going.

The purpose of diet therapy for CKD (Chronic Kidney Disease) is to treat complications (diabetes, low albumin, anemia, and fatigue to name a few), slow down the progression of the disease, and maintain a good nutritional status so if you have to start dialysis you are in the best possible nutritional shape.

WHAT STAGE OF KIDNEY DISEASE ARE YOU?

Kidney damage is graded in stages, ranging from 1 – 5, where 5 is ESRD (end stage renal disease) and means you are preparing to start dialysis so you can live without a functioning kidney. As the level goes up, the amount of functioning kidney tissue goes down. People can survive with just 10% function of their kidneys, but at that point they also usually are preparing to start dialysis. Remember, there are several options when it comes to dialysis, and you may always have the option to get on a transplant list.

Stage	Description	GFR (mL/min/1.73 m²)
1	Kidney Damage, but normal kidney function	90-130
2	Mild decrease in kidney function	60-89
3	Moderate decrease in kidney function	30-59
4	Severe decrease in kidney function (about 20% of your kidneys are functional)	15-29
5	Kidney failure, defined as end-stage renal disease, and dialysis is usually started (less than 10% of your kidneys are functional)	<15

WHAT WILL THIS BOOK TEACH YOU?

Information in this book shows you how to use food to meet your needs in your daily life. This is all about learning what a pre-dialysis kidney diet should be for your stage of kidney disease.

Overall, controlling your blood sugar if you are diabetic and blood pressure through healthy food choices and medication (if necessary) is an important part of slowing the progression of kidney disease. Diabetes and high blood pressure are the leading causes of Chronic Kidney Disease (CKD) in the United

States. Your first step is to get those conditions under control by managing your meals and having a plan.

KEYS TO THE KIDNEY DIET IN PRE-DIALYSIS

CKD is progressive in nature and happens over a longer time than we are probably aware of as part of a normal life. As your kidneys start to fail, they naturally accommodate the changes and adjust to allow you to continue to function in a normal fashion. It's only when they are heavily damaged that many people find out they have kidney disease.

> Medical Nutrition Therapy (MNT) is the use of nutrition counseling by a Registered Dietitian to help promote a medical or health goal. Many insurance companies cover MNT with a referral from a doctor. Anyone who qualifies for Medicare can receive a benefit for MNT from a Registered Dietitian with a doctor's referral to address diabetes or kidney disease. Take advantage if you have that option!

CKD is detected by two lab tests – Estimated Glomerular Filtration Rate (eGFR) and the Urine Albumin To Creatinine Ratio (UACR). The eGFR tells you what stage you are in, and your UACR tells your doctor how quickly you might progress to the next stage of kidney disease based on the amount of protein in your urine. The UACR is the preferred measure for screening, assessing, and monitoring kidney damage. A lab completes the test, and is not a urine dipstick test done in your doctor's office. Having protein in your urine, also known as albuminuria, is an independent risk factor for CKD progression in addition to your eGFR level.

The keys to the diet during the pre-dialysis stage are as follows:

- Control blood pressure by reducing the amount of sodium in the diet
- Reduce the protein intake to an appropriate level depending on nutritional status
- Managing diabetes through proper meal planning

We are not talking about potassium and phosphorus at this stage, because if you can control the sodium and protein intake in your diet, you can slow the damage and delay the need for a more restrictive diet. You should focus on improving your diet by reducing sodium and protein. If you are a diabetic, you can work on getting your hemoglobin A1C to 7.5% or below.

So, in learning about renal or kidney diets for people with pre-dialysis kidney disease, it's important to start with the general information and get more specific. I am going to lead you through this process and help you learn more about what each step means and what it will take to keep your kidneys healthy.

WHAT ARE MY LIMITATIONS?

For your personal limitations, I would recommend discussing your individual conditions with a nephrologist. This book is designed for people with pre-dialysis kidney disease in stages 1 – 4, who may also have diabetes.

The current nutritional guidelines and recommendations for management of adults with kidney disease are as follows:

STAGES 1 – 2

Follow the DASH (Dietary Approaches To Stopping Hypertension) Diet guidelines – adopt a diet that emphasizes fruits, vegetables, and low fat dairy products; include whole grains, poultry, fish, and nuts; eat only small amounts of red meats, sweets and sugar containing beverages; decrease the amounts of total and saturated fats and cholesterol as well as a modest increase in protein (1.4 gm/kg) overall. Eating 8-10 servings per day of fruits and vegetables with daily intake will decrease blood pressure and improve overall health. A reduction in dietary sodium intake lowers blood pressure as well in Chronic Kidney Disease, and you should reduce intake of high sodium foods to a total intake of 2400 mg/day of sodium.

The DASH diet contains a higher protein, potassium, and phosphorus content than recommended for patients with chronic kidney disease stages 3-4. If your GFR is below 60mL/min/1.73m², you should not follow a high protein diet such as that in a DASH diet. The DASH diet also averages about 4,500 mg/d of potassium and can cause problems in people with stages 3-4 kidney disease.

In stages 1-2, it is very important to control your related conditions – whether diabetes or high blood pressure, which slows the progression of damage to your kidneys. Additionally, with diabetes, keeping your blood sugar levels in control makes a significant difference.

STAGES 3 – 5
Protein in these stages is limited, from 0.8 gm/kg/day (grams per kilogram per day) in stage 3 to 0.6 gm/kd/day in stage 5. Protein is limited to improve symptoms of waste products in the blood and reduce related conditions. Typically there is not a fluid restriction as the kidneys are still filtering the blood and creating urine. Sodium is limited to about 1500 mg/day, and protein is between 0.6 - 0.8 g/kg/day.

Phosphorus in the diet might start to be limited if serum phosphorus is less than 4.6 mg/dL in your blood or PTH (parathyroid hormone) is elevated. Phosphorus would be limited to 800 - 1000 mg/day. If your phosphorus has not been affected, than there is no need to limit your intake. Also, potassium might be lost through the kidneys if you are on certain types of diuretics, so ask your doctor if you need to eat a higher amount of potassium. Otherwise, the need to limit nutrients is usually protein and sodium intake.

WHAT ARE CALORIES?

Calories are a unit of measure for the energy value in food. When a food has more calories, it gives you more "gas" for your tank. Your body needs that energy to work – your muscles use it, your heart uses it, and your body stores the extra energy as fat. If you lose weight, you didn't take in as many calories as your "engine" needed so it used some of your body fat or muscle to provide that energy to live. If you gain weight, you took in more calories than your body used so it stored them as fat (or muscle if you are training). Either way, your body uses calories all the time – when you do everyday things, when you exercise, and even when you are asleep.

It really is that simple. When you see a fad diet that talks about eating all protein or just cabbage soup, at the end of the day it is causing a reduction in the amount of calories you consume so you lose weight because you didn't eat as much.

Let me add to this – calories are the overall general energy that a food provides. Calories come from different places – fat, alcohol, carbohydrate and protein all contain different amounts of calories. So, when you add them together in a food, you get the total amount of calories. So, later I will be explaining about how to decide how much of each type of food to eat, but for now, it's about calories. Once you know the calorie amounts, you can move into dividing it out into types of calories – from carbohydrate, protein, or fat.

How Many Calories Should I Eat?

Now, you are probably wondering how many calories you should eat. Since that determines whether you lose or gain weight, it can be a very important question.

How many calories you need in a day is based on your age and how active you are. If you are active, you need more calories because you are using them up. If you are inactive, you need less.

You can calculate your calorie needs using an equation called a Basal Metabolic Rate (BMR) formula.

If you are overweight, you need to know your adjusted body weight (ABW). You need to calculate the amount of "active" tissue weight in your body, so you will have to make some adjustments to the number for your weight that you use in calculations.

Some of your extra weight is active muscle tissue, yet the majority is fat which does not consume a lot of additional calories. The weight that you will use in the calculations is called an ABW since it accounts for your extra weight that needs more calories.

One more example to ensure you understand why you need to adjust the weight – if you used your current weight, the amount of calories would be way too high for what your body is actually using and you would gain a lot of weight. If you used just the normal body weight, then you will have too few calories and that causes you to be very hungry and your body often slows down the metabolic rate when you are not eating enough. So it works the opposite of what you might expect it to.

Use the following tables to determine your healthy body weight.

For women and men, you should add 1 inch to your height to be on the right line. Now, it does refer to different size frames for men and women. I think if you are "large boned" you know it. But for most people, they are in the medium frame range. So I would recommend using the medium frame if you are not sure where to start.

If you are overweight according to the chart, you should do the following to calculate your adjusted body weight.

Take your current weight, subtract your ideal weight (weight from chart) and take that number times .25. Then you add the number you came up with to your ideal body weight number. This accounts for the energy that your additional weight needs to function. It's a low number because most of your extra weight is usually fat.

Step 1: Calculate your adjusted body weight using the information provided at this point if you need to. (I will show you the calculation in the next step).

WOMEN				MEN			
Height	**Frame Size**			**Height**	**Frame Size**		
Ft. In.	**Small**	**Med.**	**Large**	**Ft. In.**	**Small**	**Med.**	**Large**
4'10"	102-111	109-121	118-131	5'2"	128-134	131-141	138-150
4'11"	103-113	111-123	120-134	5'3"	130-136	133-143	140-153
5'0"	104-115	113-126	122-137	5'4"	132-138	135-145	142-156
5'1"	106-118	115-129	125-140	5'5"	134-140	137-148	144-160
5'2"	108-121	118-132	128-143	5'6"	136-142	139-151	146-164
5'3"	111-124	121-135	131-147	5'7"	138-145	142-154	149-168
5'4"	114-127	124-138	134-151	5'8"	140-148	145-157	152-172
5'5"	117-130	127-141	137-155	5'9"	142-151	156-160	155-176
5'6"	120-133	130-144	140-159	5'10"	144-154	151-163	158-180
5'7"	123-136	133-144	143-163	5'11"	146-157	154-166	161-184
5'8"	126-139	136-150	146-167	6'0"	149-160	157-170	164-188
5'9"	129-142	139-153	149-170	6'1"	152-164	160-174	168-192
5'10"	132-145	142-156	152-173	6'2"	155-168	165-178	172-197
5'11"	135-148	145-159	155-176	6'3"	158-172	167-182	176-202
6'0"	138-151	148-162	158-176	6'4"	162-176	171-187	181-207

Step 2. Now, you can **calculate your calorie needs using the BMR equations**. Enter your adjusted body weight (as your weight) you just calculated if you are overweight – or use your normal body weight if you are not overweight.

English BMR Formula

Women: BMR = 655 + (4.35 x weight in pounds) + (4.7 x height in inches) - (4.7 x age in years)

Men: BMR = 66 + (6.23 x weight in pounds) + (12.7 x height in inches) - (6.8 x age in year)

Metric BMR Formula

Women: BMR = 655 + (9.6 x weight in kilos) + (1.8 x height in cm) - (4.7 x age in years)

Men: BMR = 66 + (13.7 x weight in kilos) + (5 x height in cm) - (6.8 x age in years)

So, to complete an example for you for a man and a woman:

Woman: Age 60, 5' 3" tall (including 1 inch for height chart), weight 220 pounds. Her ideal weight is: 128 pounds. (I took the middle of the medium range).

So – 220 pounds – 128 pounds = 92 pounds x .25 = 23 pounds. Add that amount to ideal weight: 128 +

23= 151 pounds to use in calculations – including information about how much protein to eat.

Man: Age 60, 6'2" tall (including 1 inch height for the height chart), weight 250 pounds. His ideal weight is: 172 pounds. (I took the middle of the medium range).

So – 250 pounds – 172 pounds = 78 pounds x .25 = 19.5 pounds. Add that amount to ideal weight: 172 pounds + 19.5 pounds = 192 pounds (rounded up) to use in calculations for calories and protein amounts.

Now, let's calculate their calorie needs so we can figure out how much to feed them, using equation from box above. I will round up or down the decimal points in case you are wondering where they are going.

Woman: 655+ (4.35 x 151 pounds) + (4.7 x 63 inches) – (4.7 x 60 years old) =

655 + 657 + 296 – 282 = 1326 calories for the day

Man: 66 + (6.23 x 192 pounds) + (12.7 x 74 inches) – (6.8 x 60 years old) =

66 + 1196 + 940 – 408 = 1794 calories for the day

(I hope this helps you be able to figure your own calorie needs)

Remember, these calculations are not exact but are a good number for you to use. Based on your activity level and amount of muscle weight, you could need a higher number of calories.

Step 3. The basic calorie number is the number that you need to lay in bed and rest all day. So you need to multiply the calorie number you just calculated by 1.1 – 1.5 depending on your activity level. This will be a judgment call on your part, but you should add some for activity. If you find you are losing weight, you will want to add calories to make sure you are at the right amount of calories you need to maintain your weight.

You need to find a balance if you are trying to lose weight with a calorie level that allows you to lose 1-2 pounds per week. If you lose faster than that, you might be losing muscle mass which is not a good thing.

My sample man and woman are walking 30 minutes 3 days a week and still work full time jobs. Therefore, I am going to give them an activity factor of 1.2.

Final calorie levels:

Woman: 1326 x 1.2 = 1591 calories

Man: 1794 x 1.2 = 2153 calories for the day.

[Use your judgment about which number is best for you]

Now, in order to figure out how many calories you are eating every day, you have to track them. You need to write down the foods and serving sizes and calorie information for the foods you are eating every day so you know how much you eat. You don't remember all the things that you consumed this morning let alone yesterday – plus you have to add your beverages. I would recommend starting with a lined paper notepad, and write down the items you eat along with calories, protein and sodium amounts.

Keep your diary or food record for everything you eat over the next few days, and it will surprise you. Especially when you have to count everything that goes into your mouth that is food (gum usually not included). Make sure you document the amounts of food eaten as well as the amounts of liquid consumed. Even if it's water, so you can determine if you need to change any behaviors.

Remember, in your case, all solid and liquid intake matters. All of the foods you eat contribute to your health, and you should make healthy choices to improve your kidney function. You feel better when you are eating well. Also, pay attention to your timing of meals and your portions. You can use smaller plates and eat slowly to keep your portion sizes in control if that helps you.

Step 4. Calculating the amount of protein you need to consume.

If you are in stages 1-2, eating according to the DASH diet plan and being healthier with exercise will improve your health and likely slow your progression of kidney disease. But in stage 3-5, you need to figure out the amount of protein to eat for the day and track it so you are not eating too much.

For most people with kidney disease at stage 3 or 4, you are in need of about 0.8 gm of protein per kilogram. As your kidney disease worsens, you should lower that amount of protein even more – into the 0.7 gm/kg range or 0.6 gm/kg. This amount of protein is considered adequate to improve your health but reduce your kidney failure symptoms.

To calculate the amount of protein that you need, divide your weight in pounds by 2.2, then multiply that number X 0.8 = the grams of protein you need to eat in a day. Earlier in this document, when you calculated your ideal weight (if you are considered overweight), that is the number you should use to calculate your protein intake needs.

For example:

A person weighs 150 pounds. 150 / 2.2 = 68.2 kg

Then you take 68.2 kg X 0.8 = 54.5 grams of protein for the day

One ounce of meat contains approximately 7 gm of protein – so this person can have about 8 ounces of meat for the day (7.8 to be exact). Now, don't forget, many foods contain protein and you need to read labels – lots of starches and carbohydrates contain small amounts of protein. So, you would likely just need to count the amount of protein on labels. That will keep you in the "safe" zone. Or try to maintain eating only about 6 ounces in actual meat and consider the rest to come from "other" sources – vegetables, dairy, fruits, grains, beans and nuts.

READING FOOD LABELS IS A VERY IMPORTANT SKILL TO DEVELOP

You will notice quickly when you are tracking your own food that you rely on the food labels to tell you a lot of information. You might not be able to determine the amount of potassium and phosphorus in the food, but you can find out the big things like calories, servings, serving size, and amount of macronutrients (carbohydrate, protein, and fat) in the USA.

When you have chronic kidney disease, you have a need to limit some nutrients in your diet. You should be aware of the amount of sodium, phosphorus, or potassium a food contains. Limiting fats, such as saturated fats and trans fats, are important due to the higher risk of cardiovascular disease that you have.

[A good place on the web with information about food labels is at:
http://www.fda.gov/food/ResourcesForYou/Consumers/NFLPM/ucm274593.htm]

Reviewing the food label, you can see how many servings are in the container and how much is a serving. Make sure you know how to portion out this food product. This product has 2 servings in the container, so eating all of the food in the container in one sitting would require you to multiply the totals in the other areas by 2 to get the true amount of calories, fat, and protein. It very clearly states that you should eat about 1 cup for one serving.

In that serving, you get 280 calories, 660 mg of sodium and 5 gm of protein. As far as the daily value column, you can see that it tells you the percentage of the total daily allowance this serving contains. A daily serving of sodium is about 2,400 mg of sodium, which is a low amount of sodium for the average American diet. If the daily value says 5% or less, it is considered low in that nutrient. If it has 20% or more, it is considered high. This product is high for sodium content, and should be a food that you eat less often. And don't forget that's just for one serving.

Sometimes, the nutrition facts label will list sodium, potassium, and phosphorus. Manufacturer's do not have to list potassium and phosphorus. This means you need to look at the ingredients listing for more clues about how much potassium or phosphorus it might contain. Many products have added phosphate, as well as naturally occurring phosphorus. Read the ingredients listing for the word phosphorus or PHOS on the ingredient listing. You also need to look for the word potassium in the food listing as well. Many of the chemicals used to preserve foods contain phosphorus and potassium and add to the total amount in these foods. Potassium chloride might be used in place of sodium chloride to reduce the overall sodium in a product.   See the picture of an ingredient

Ingredients: Potatoes*, Modified Corn Starch, Maltodextrin, Salt, Sugar, Roasted Garlic*, Mono and Diglycerides, Nonfat Milk, Natural Flavor, Yeast Extract, Parsley Flakes, Spice, Potassium Phosphate, Color Added. Freshness Preserved by Sodium Bisulfite, Citric Acid. *Dried
CONTAINS MILK; MAY CONTAIN WHEAT AND SOY INGREDIENTS.

listing with potassium and phosphate highlighted.

Finally, I want to remind you that foods are listed on the ingredient panel in order of the amount in the food by weight.   The food has the most of the first product (in this case – potatoes) and the least of the last food (in this case – citric acid).

Claims on food packages can help you identify healthier alternatives as well.   If a label on a food contains the words: saturated fat free, low saturated fat, less saturated fat, and trans fat free, those items are better for you to eat when you need to lower the amount of saturated and trans fats in your diet.   If you need to lower the sodium in your diet, you should look for foods with the terms: sodium free, very low sodium, low sodium and reduced salt – but be aware that they may replace sodium with potassium and always read your ingredients sections as well as the nutrition facts labels.

Right now, you should focus on understanding the portion size and amounts of protein and sodium per portion.   In addition, if you have diabetes, you will want to understand and limit the total carbohydrate in the food you eat.

Now That You Know How Much To Eat, Do You Need To Gain Weight?

You usually will be aware of your need to gain weight. If you need to know, ask your doctor. As your kidney disease progresses, you might not feel like eating. You must keep your protein and nutritional status in good standing so your health is not compromised in the long term – with kidney dialysis you need to have your albumin levels above 3.9 to improve your outcomes over the long term.

If you need to gain weight, or eat more, then you can increase the calories in the foods you already are eating or you can eat more food. If you have a limited appetite because of the stage of your kidney disease or inability to control your intake, you can do some things to improve your intake. It's very important how much your protein intake is – that is a huge determination in your success with kidney disease – it makes you feel better when you have that in the right place.

Many times as your kidneys deteriorate, your appetite starts to decrease. You have many waste products building up in your blood stream and they make you feel tired and weak. Eating a better diet will help you have less waste in your blood and help your kidney function to improve and for you to feel better. But you also need to take in more calories so you have the energy to do the things you need to do.

Let me give you some ideas about how to improve your intake:

1. Eat 6 smaller meals instead of 3 larger ones. You can graze all day, or take "snacks" with you to eat – like crackers or a bar – and that will help you get more intake without stuffing it in at meals and feeling like you will burst.

2. Take a bigger portion of the foods that you know you like and feel in the mood for. If you really like rice, and you don't feel like eating the other things on your plate, go ahead and eat more rice. It will give you the energy and calories you need.

3. Try some of the foods cold instead of hot. For example, eating bread or biscuits cold might taste good to you. Or cold chicken sometimes is a great snack. Just try it.

4. Use meats that are sliced very thin – you can eat smaller amounts of them throughout the day without over doing it on the protein side.

5. Eat breads that are more thickly sliced – you can get some tasty breads as well like sourdough.

6. Eat more servings of the breads, pastas and rice to get the calories without increasing the amount of protein too much – and dip them in olive oil or use a healthy spread. (This could change if you are diabetic – watch the amount of carbohydrate in foods)

7. You can use more of the heart healthy fats like canola and olive oil or mayonnaise to increase calories without increasing protein or potassium.

8. Eating some hard candies, jellybeans, marshmallows, or chewy fruit flavored candies for snacks and desserts. Again, watch this if

you are a diabetic because of the amount of carbohydrate.

9. Cook foods in a way that adds calories – like sautéing in olive oil.

10. Drink fluids that have calories – juices and clear carbonated beverages instead of plain water or coffee. Do not do this if you are a diabetic – it will add calories and increase your blood sugar.

11. Choose foods that are easy to chew – like meatloaf, casseroles or omelets instead of hard to chew foods like steaks.

12. Add extra calories to the foods you already eat – use olive oil, mayonnaise, salad dressings, sour cream and butters.

13. Drink fluids after a meal instead of with a meal so you don't get filled up as easily with your beverages.

Fruity Frozen Dessert Recipe

Makes 5, 4-oz servings with 8 gm protein per serving

Blend the following ingredients together –

½-cup protein powder, ½-teaspoon vanilla, ½-cup hot water, and ½ cup drained regular or low sugar canned peaches. Once that is blenderized, spoon in 4 ounces Cool Whip Lite or Sugar Free, and mix by hand until blended well. Divide into individual servings in paper cups or other containers, and freeze.

Remember these ideas are helpful to improve your overall calories, and somewhat to increase protein. However, if you are in stage 3 – 5 Chronic Kidney Disease, you may not want to increase your protein. So focus on the things that talk about adding sides

Fruit Smoothie

For 2 servings (5 gm protein per serving with the protein powder, 2 gm per serving without protein powder)

½ cup fresh or frozen whole strawberries

1 cup **unfortified** rice milk

4 teaspoons sugar or sugar substitute

2 Tablespoons protein powder (optional)

Blenderize all ingredients well, pour into cups, and enjoy. If you want to save one for later, put it in a cup and freeze it.

and leaving the extra meat out. You need to get an overall number of calories as well as protein.

If your albumin level is low or your nutritional status is poor, you may need to add protein to your diet in strategic ways so that you are not overwhelmed but able to get the additional nutrition you need. Ask your doctor to be sure if you need to add more protein.

You can get some ideas about how to add protein to your diet if you need to improve your nutritional status in the information below:

1. Use a protein powder that is whey based. It is easier to digest and can be added to many regular and sugar free foods like pudding, cream pie fillings, applesauce, milk, fruit juice or soups.

2. Mix 1-2 tablespoons of the whey protein powder with a little water and make a paste. Then add it to the recipe you are making. Start adding it to some sweets to see if the taste is noticeable. You may find you can only add a

bit to the foods before you notice, but you should continue to make an effort to get the extra protein if you need it.

OR DO YOU NEED TO LOSE WEIGHT?

When you need to lose weight, you can do many things as well. It's important to understand that fad diets won't work for you most of the time. You will only regain the weight and possibly cause more problems for yourself. Choosing diets that are high in protein will further aggravate your condition, and cause further damage to your kidneys. And diets that are high protein are going to be hard on your kidneys and increase the rate of damage so you will possibly get to dialysis sooner.

You might need to lose weight to get on the transplant list, or you might just need to be healthier. (If you need to lose weight but still improve your protein levels, look at some of the ideas for adding protein powder to your meals above).

Think about what has worked for you in the past when you lost weight. The truth about losing weight (whether you want to hear it or not) is that calories in vs. calories out is the right way to lose weight. So, taking in less calories than your body uses for the day creates a deficit that will help you lose weight. You are not going to lose the weight overnight – you didn't gain it that quickly (even though it feels like it). If you can exercise – get a plan together and do it. Something as simple as 30 minutes of walking every night or morning will make a big difference in your health. If you can't walk, go to the library, rent a DVD with chair exercises, and get started. You can exercise in a wheel chair or sitting down.

WAYS TO DECREASE YOUR OVERALL CALORIES

Ok, so here are some ideas about how to decrease your overall calories. Remember – take in less than you use for calories. Find a way to exercise every day.

1. Order your salad dressing on the side. You can dip your fork into the dressing. Even better – use balsamic vinegar and olive oil, with just a bit of oil and a lot of vinegar to make your salad extra tasty. Use fresh ground pepper to improve the taste.

2. When you make gravies and soups, chill them to have the fat rise to the top and you can remove it before you eat.

3. Follow a meal plan that divides the meals up into reasonable amounts and makes it easy to understand. It's as simple as putting things together for a meal, and you use your choices to build the meal. You also have room for snacks.

4. Buy the lean cuts of meat and hamburger. You don't get to eat much protein – especially from animal sources, so get a great cut of meat or 95% lean hamburger.

5. Roast, broil or grill your meats to make them less fatty. The fat drips off and you have a leaner meal.

6. Take out one serving of your higher calorie side dishes – breads, chips, crackers. Count out or weigh the items. Then put away the package. You can have that taste and not keep getting more from the package.

7. Eat all your food mindfully. You should stop, sit calmly, think about the food and savor the taste of the food. Don't sit at your desk and work or sit in front of the TV and eat. Pay attention to your food and enjoy it.

8. Think about whether or not you are actually hungry when you are eating. If you are not at least somewhat hungry, then get up and go for a walk instead. Or a change of scenery. You will be pleasantly surprised at how quickly the feeling goes away.

9. Have just one cookie. Or a small piece of cake. You can head off the binge many times with just a taste of the food. What you don't realize is, eating more chocolate doesn't improve the taste. The first bites are the best ones – so stop after you have had a couple of bites and put the food down. If you are eating slowly, you will be able to savor the taste.

10. Plan to have "dessert" once a week. As a matter of fact, stop thinking about dessert as a sweet, and eat a low phosphorus or potassium fruit for dessert every day.

11. Bake items that you previously fried – onion rings, French fries, chicken and fish. Just spray them with a little cooking spray, and bake them at a slightly higher temperature to get them crispy.

12. Instead of making creamed, au gratin or scalloped vegetables – steam, stew or boil them. Season them with some salt free seasoning, like vinegar or lemon juice.

13. Drink water instead of beverages with calories like soda and juices.

14. Make your sandwiches with mostly lettuce, cucumber, and other vegetables and add a little bit of meat. That way you are making a low protein sandwich as well.
15. Make your casseroles with smaller pieces of meat and add in extra vegetables to make them filling yet lower in calories.
16. Your plate can be 75% vegetables and starches and just 25% or less meat or chicken. That way you are not adding the extra calories and fat from meat and you are eating lower protein.

The best thing that you can do is follow a meal plan and a pattern with information about what you need to eat and how to make the recipes. You need to understand that you can eat some of a lot of foods. If your world is very black and white regarding what you eat – can't have this or only can have that – you will get bored quickly. As long as you are holding steady or making progress on your kidney disease, you are doing fine. But eliminating an entire group of foods – potatoes, milk, etc – makes for a very bland diet. You have to live with this diet for the rest of your life. I want you to succeed, so do not eliminate everything – yet. Unless your doctor says so. Listen to them, because I don't know all your specific condition issues.

General Information About Macro Nutrients You Need To Know

The shared part of food is calories. All food has calories. Not all food has the same amount of calories, so you have to know some information about what macro nutrients are and how they affect your kidney diet. Sure, it sounds like a lot of work, but it's ok – you are going to understand how the diet works by the time we are done.

Carbohydrates

Carbohydrates are the main source of calories in most diets. It is recommended that you eat 50-60% of their calories from carbohydrates. Carbohydrates (carbs or CHO) are made from simple sugars or starches, and are broken down in your digestive system into sugar for your body to use as fuel. Carbs are also part of whole grains and whole wheat foods, and fiber is "technically" considered carbohydrate.

Some carbohydrates are absorbed faster – simple sugars. Some examples of simple sugars are white or brown sugar, honey, syrup, fruit sugars, and milk sugar (lactose). Most of the simple sugars are pure carbohydrate and don't contribute a lot of nutritional value to a diet. If you are not diabetic and you need to increase your calories, simple sugars in the form of candies can be a good way to add calories.

Other types of carbohydrates are not as easily absorbed and provide a little more "full" feeling when eaten. These are called complex carbohydrates, and are foods like breads, pastas and grains. Beans also contain complex carbohydrate and protein. Complex carbohydrates also break down into sugars, but at a slower rate. They typically contain more vitamins, minerals and fiber so they are considered more "nutritious". Foods that are considered complex carbohydrates are breads, pastas, cereals, rice, fruits, vegetables, and whole grain products. Diets that include whole grains as the main form of carbohydrates, an abundance of fruits and vegetables, and a good variety of omega-3 rich foods provide significant protection from kidney damage.

Now, if you have diabetes, you will likely already know about carbohydrate as it is the food that raises your blood sugar levels. The amount of carbohydrate in your food and how quickly it is released are important factors in how the food is used by our body for fuel. The term for how quickly a food is absorbed in the blood stream is called the glycemic index. You want to eat low glycemic index foods if you are a diabetic. Carbohydrates with lots of fiber, like beans, whole grains, and oatmeal doesn't get broken down as quickly and are low on the glycemic index scale. White bread, plain pasta, candies and plain white rice are high glycemic index foods because they are absorbed quickly. Eat less of the high glycemic index foods to help with diabetes.

Food labels have listings of the amount of carbohydrate in one serving. As we discussed before in the nutrition facts labels section, it is very important to understand how much is a serving and how much of each type of nutrient it contains.

FATS – SATURATED AND UNSATURATED

Fats can be good for you. As a matter of fact, with kidney disease, a fat can be a source of calories that you don't have to worry that it contains extra protein or phosphorus. They provide energy and calories without a lot of extra stuff we don't need. Now, if you are trying to lose weight, you will be watching your fat closely. But if you are trying to gain weight, fats can be your friend. Just choose the best types. It is recommended to consume 30% or less of your calories from fat, and less than 10% from saturated fats. You should also review cholesterol and only consume about 200 mg of cholesterol or less daily. That will probably be easier on a low protein diet. Cholesterol is part of all animal foods, and when you eat less protein, you eat less cholesterol.

The best fats for you to use are the following:

> Olive Oil (use for dressing and dipping)
> Canola Oil
> Sesame Oil (very flavorful)
> Fatty Fish (salmon, tuna, herring)
> Safflower or Sunflower Oil
> Corn, Cottonseed, or Soybean Oil

You might eat more fat than you should. It's very easy to do. Your body naturally uses fat as to insulate your organs, to provide you with energy, and to help with absorbing some vitamins. But since you have kidney failure, you also have a higher risk of developing heart disease. So, it is important to eat the right kinds of fats. Fats that are considered heart healthy fats, like unsaturated fats.

Fats that are liquid at room temperature are unsaturated fats. These are healthier for you than fats that are solid at room temperature – also known as saturated fats. A good way to remember which is which is to recall that if they are solid at room temperature – that is how they will be in your arteries. So, a stick of butter will be solid in your arteries, and you really don't want solid fat in your blood vessels. Liquid (unsaturated) fats will remain in liquid form in your body and allow you to benefit from their heart healthy properties. They do not form artery-clogging plaques that can cause damage to your blood vessels and heart. It's best to eat more of the unsaturated fats – so given a choice between dipping your bread in oil and spreading butter on it – choose the oil.

When I was teaching cholesterol lowering classes, I found that patients who eat a diet low in saturated fat (20 gm or less per day) reduced their total cholesterol and LDL numbers better than those who didn't. Labels show the amount of total fat and the amount of saturated fat in the food (and usually the amount of trans-fat). You will be able to track this amount daily in your records and improve your overall health by lowering the amount of saturated and trans-fat you eat.

In choosing foods that are healthy for your heart, you can do the following things to lower your intake of fats:

➢ Grill, broil, bake, roast, or stir-fry foods instead of deep frying
➢ Cook with non-stick cooking spray or a small amount of olive oil instead of butter

> Trim fat from meats and remove skin from poultry before eating
> Choose lean cuts of meat – like loin or round
> Eat more fish
> Eat beans if you don't have to limit your phosphorus
> Use more whole fruits and vegetables in your cooking
> Eat lowfat milk, yogurt and cheeses

PROTEINS – BEEF, CHICKEN, TURKEY, FISH?

Now, the last "macro" nutrient is the protein category. Learning what foods are in this category can be somewhat obvious, but protein is contained in many foods so as a person with kidney disease, you need to pay attention to your food labels. You should aim to consume about 10% of your calories from protein in stages 3 & 4. This may be significantly less than you are used to eating. But it has been proven over and over that lowering the protein in your diet in pre-dialysis kidney disease reduces symptoms and can extend the time your kidneys function prior to starting dialysis.

Protein is used in your body to build healthy muscles, bones, hair and skin. Each cell of your body is made from protein pieces (building blocks) called amino acids. Your body breaks down protein that you eat into amino acids to use to build and repair your muscles and organs in your body. Some amino acids are known as essential amino acids because your body cannot make them (like it can make so many other hormones and amino acids you need). They are essential because you must consume foods with these amino acids in them for your body to have to use.

So, you need protein. Now your kidneys are having a tough time dealing with protein, so you have to make some changes.

You see, as your body breaks down protein, you produce byproducts that are known as urea or uric acid. One of the measures of your health is the BUN (blood urea nitrogen – I talk more about labs in another book). The more urea and uric acid in your blood, the more your health suffers. And urea is excreted from your body through urine created by your kidneys. Therefore, the less functional your kidneys are, the more urea builds up in your blood and makes you feel poorly. That is why we recommend you eat less protein – so you get what your body needs but not so much that your kidneys are struggling to remove the waste products from your blood.

Proteins are sometimes referred to as animal or vegetable proteins, or high biological value (HBV) or low biological value (LBV) proteins. Proteins with more of the essential amino acids are considered HBV proteins. Mainly, these are from animal sources. Animal protein is easier for your body to use. It's important to eat the majority of your protein from HBV sources so your body can easily use them for replacement in your body. (Note that dairy products are high in phosphorus, so if you need to limit phosphorus you might have to use less of it to control your overall limits). As a diabetic, you should be aware that protein does not contain carbohydrate and therefore does not increase your blood sugar levels.

High Biological Value Proteins

- ✓ Beef, pork, and lamb
- ✓ Chicken, turkey, and other poultry
- ✓ Eggs
- ✓ Fish, shrimp and other seafood
- ✓ Dairy products
- ✓ Soy (tofu, edamame)

Low Biological Value Proteins

- ✓ Nuts
- ✓ Dried Beans and Peas
- ✓ Some grains – amaranth, buckwheat, quinoa, brown rice and rye

EATING THE RIGHT AMOUNT OF PROTEIN

Your goal should be to eat the "right" amount of protein. Not too much and not too little. It is common for people with kidney disease to lose their desire for protein type of foods, and have difficulty getting enough protein. That is why you need to know how much to get and how you are going to ensure your body gets the right amount of protein. If it sounds complicated, it is not.

You may be thinking that you are not going to feel very full without eating more protein. Some ideas that will help you to feel more full are:

- ✓ Add rice or pasta to your soups to increase the bulk without adding much protein or phosphorus
- ✓ Use milk substitutes (like non-dairy creamer or rice milk) when making cream soups
- ✓ Use vegetables and grains as the main part of the dish, with a smaller piece of HBV protein

- ✓ Cut meat into smaller pieces and use in casseroles with rice or pasta
- ✓ Make a chef salad, but use lots of lettuce and vegetables with a little bit of meats, cheese, and eggs
- ✓ Use a stronger flavored cheese – sharp cheddar for example, to give a stronger flavor with less of the actual product

Following a well planned, low protein diet is the key to slowing the progression of kidney disease, reducing the risk of anorexia, and delay the onset of uremia (failure of the kidneys which leads to dialysis). It is well documented that people who follow a low protein diet, as long as they are eating the proper amount of calories, improve in their nutritional status. Following a protein restricted diet reduces the symptoms of people with kidney disease and allows them to continue to live a full and prosperous life.

How big is an ounce of meat, or 3 ounces? Serving sizes of protein can be difficult to estimate. It's important to know, especially if you are out to eat or at a friend's house. When you are trying to gauge the number of ounces in a meat product, you should realize that a matchbook sized portion is about 1 ounce, and a deck of cards is about 3 ounces (or the palm of your hand – usually).

Not getting enough protein can lead to other problems, and makes you less healthy to start dialysis if you need to. You might feel more fatigue, get more infections, and lose weight. Ask your doctor about your nutritional status – either through your albumin levels or your other labs. It is important that you know your status so you can be aware when it changes. With albumin, the normal level is around 4 grams per deciliter (4.0 g/dL).

WATER – HOW MUCH?

Water is key to any diet, but many people on a kidney diet know that water can be a very significant part of their diet. Unless your doctor tells you to restrict your fluid intake, you should make every effort to drink as much fluid as normal.

Why? Because being well hydrated when your kidneys are still working is important to allowing them to do their natural functioning. They have to work harder when you don't have enough fluid in your body. If your urine is dark, you should concentrate on drinking more fluid. You are likely dehydrated.

How much water – good question! If you listen to many people, it's 64 ounces per day. A good average amount is about 1 – 2 quarts per day (32 - 64 ounces). But your body should also be creating about that amount of urine. Therefore, if you are not and are retaining water, you need to discuss with your doctor. Food also has water in it, so you get water from the food you eat.

If you have light colored urine, you are likely drinking enough water/fluids. Since this book is about pre-dialysis kidney failure, your kidneys should be working. Realize that you will have a limitation when you are on dialysis, but not usually until the later stages of kidney failure (stage 5 normally).

Fluid status affects your laboratory values, so make sure you are fully hydrated prior to having labs drawn or your creatinine can be measured incorrectly.

WHAT DO I DO TO FOLLOW A RENAL DIABETIC DIET?

So let's think about this. You may have had diabetes for a while, most likely. You have learned about what carbohydrates are and how to eat them. Now, even if you were following a strict diabetes diet, and doing your best to manage your blood sugars you can get kidney problems. It seems to be an almost inevitable part of things. SO don't beat yourself up about it.

The amount of carbohydrate you eat affects how well you control your diabetes. When you limit your carbohydrates (bread, sweets, pasta, rice, potatoes, and starchy vegetables), you automatically increase the amount of protein and fat that you eat. As your diabetes knowledge has improved, you are eating less bread and pasta on your diabetic diet to keep your blood sugar down. Carbohydrate is found in both pasta, grains, sugars, desserts and some "vegetables": - corn, peas, and potatoes come to mind. These are mainly starch and contain little fiber.

Your diet can be improved some by eating less of the highly refined grains, and more of the whole grain products out there. They are also known as unrefined grains. I realize that you may have been told not to eat whole grain bread, but in this case, unless you are having a lot of problems with potassium, you can eat whole grains. Unrefined grains are the items labeled whole grains, whole wheat and they contain fiber. Fiber is good for you. You can eat fiber and it does not break down into sugars that are absorbed by your blood stream when you are trying to follow a healthy renal diabetic diet.

You have learned to adapt and eat less carbohydrate. You are keeping your blood sugars below the 150's and feel good, right? You can't drink regular sugary sodas (clear nor not). You are portioning your food out – using the label information or measurement to attain the right amount of carbohydrate at that meal. You can balance out the amount of food that you eat through the day to be healthier.

A RENAL DIABETIC DIET TAKES INTO ACCOUNT BOTH CARBOHYDRATE AND PROTEIN

You know that carbohydrate is what affects your blood sugar, and you have learned to eat the higher quality (more nutritious) carbohydrates – those higher in fiber and more complex carbohydrates. Have you filled in the missing amounts with protein and fat? Fat does not raise your blood sugar in the same way that glucose (sugar) does. It may, over time, be broken down into sugar for your body, but it's much easier for your body to store it – a simple reason why you should try not to eat a ton of it.

In the past, you possibly used protein to fill in for the missing parts of your meal – it doesn't add carbohydrate and increase your blood sugar, yet it keeps you feeling full. If your body wants to use protein for energy, you have to break it down and that uses some energy. So it's less likely to be used as fuel for your body. That was great, wasn't it?

Now, you have kidney disease. That means you have to watch the amount of protein that you eat. ARGH!

So, protein is in a lot of foods. Protein is (obviously) meats, pork, chicken, veal, and turkey. Protein is also a part of many carbohydrate foods as well. It's in bread, vegetables, milk, cheese and a lot of other things. Learning to cut back some will be helpful to your kidney failure. You know you need to do this – it won't be too hard.

As your kidney failure worsens (I hope it doesn't but it might), you eat less protein until you are in end stage renal disease (ESRD) – then the protein increases. But for now, you will need to follow the recommendations made earlier in the book for the stage of kidney failure that you are in. Your kidneys are sensitive to protein, and you would do best to eat a higher percentage of the high biological value protein but less protein overall.

Think about what you need to eat. Are you a small meals eater? Do you eat breakfast? Do you eat a large meal at lunch? What are your favorite foods? I ask because the best meal plan is the meal plan that you will follow. If you want smaller meals throughout the day – structure your meals that way.

START OUT THINKING LIKE A DIABETIC

As a diabetic, you should understand how many calories you need to eat. Earlier in this book we calculated the amount of calories that you need for a day. If your blood sugars are still high with that number, you can decrease it some. But don't starve yourself. So let's say you need 1700 calories per day for your meal plan. This means that if you like to eat 3 meals and a snack, you will now divide that up through the day.

Save about 200 calories for your snack. That makes it 1500 calories for the day. Then you can eat 3 500 calorie meals, or two 250 calorie meals, and one 1000 calorie meal plus a snack. Or however that works for your day. If you like big breakfast and small lunches, work it that way.

You might be wondering, how do I know I am eating 250 calories. Stick to reading labels – most foods have one. If you search out recipes on line, you can find the carbohydrate and calories for the serving. Write it down and know what you are planning to eat.

Of the 1700 calories, you should aim for 40-50% from carbohydrate – so in this case you take 850 calories (50%) as carbohydrate. 850 calories equals how many grams of carbohydrate, you ask? 1 gram of carbohydrate equals 4 calories – so it's easy to divide it out – 850/4 = 212.5 grams of carbohydrate for the day. Divide that up for the day as part of your meals – again so it matches your desired plan for the day. (I'm going to give you an easier way to divide this up in a moment)

Now, that you kind of know how you want to spread out your meals with both calories and carbohydrates – what goes in each meal?

NOW THINK ABOUT YOUR RENAL PART OF THE DIET

So, you know how much carbohydrate and how many calories and how many meals per day you are going to eat. Good.

Think now about the protein restriction, and then needing to combine it with the other restrictions. I know right about now it's getting confusing.

Use your hand, and not just to move the fork between your plate and your mouth. You can use your hand to make a healthy meal that is right for both diabetes and renal disease. Your palm is about the size of a 3 ounce portion of meat. 3 ounces is 21 grams of protein. That should be about right for your meal. When you are in stages 3 & 4, 6-8 ounces of meat per day should be ok. Remember you are also getting protein from other foods.

Now for the amount of carbohydrate for the meal. Eat 3-4 servings (your fingers can help you remember to eat no more than four). One serving of carbohydrate is 15 gm of carbohydrate – so you can eat 45-60 grams of carbohydrate per meal. Again, eating more fiber and whole grain products helps keep your blood sugar low. Your body absorbs them more slowly and releases insulin at a slower pace so it can use the carbohydrate in the foods over time and not give you as much of a spike in blood sugar levels.

Think about the types of fruits and vegetables that you can eat. As a renal patient, you should really limit certain types of fruits and vegetables because of the amount of potassium in them. You should eat more of the whole fruits and vegetables (that have more fiber than processed ones) – apples, blackberries, grapes, mandarin oranges, peaches, pineapple, strawberries. Eat more asparagus, green or wax beans, cucumber, mushrooms, peppers, lettuce and zucchini. Remember – the fruits count as carbohydrate servings but the vegetables do not. Load up on your vegetables and count portion sizes on your fruits.

Most of the time, you can eat small amounts of even high potassium foods because you are not over indulging. Your body can handle some potassium, just not too much at one time. So if you want to have an occasional tomato or potato, no one is stopping you. Potatoes do count as a carbohydrate serving, so you have to keep within your limit for the meal. I know many people say – I can't have potatoes – but you can have a small amount unless your doctor says absolutely not. I am not an all or nothing person – I believe that you can fit the foods you want to eat into this diet – just not too much.

Eat more often from the whole grain carbohydrates that are not as high in potassium, like brown rice and noodles that are whole grain. You can buy quick cooking brown rice, and have it as part of your meals much more easily. Still watch your portion size.

PUTTING THEM TOGETHER

You take the carbohydrates and add some protein. But what about fat? You need to add some fat to your meal to make you feel fuller. Add a tsp of butter to your bread, or use oil – even better. And use vinegar and oil salad dressing to have a low sodium dressing that is also low carbohydrate.

Fat is needed, but you might be eating too much. Watch out for saturated fats, and stick to below 20 gm of saturated or trans fat per day. And make it stick to within your total calories for the day and meal.

Calories are really the key to keeping you at a healthy weight. That and exercise.

Serving Sizes Review

Here are some general guidelines about how much a portion is for many of the typical foods you eat daily.

1 bagel or roll = 6 ounce can of tuna

1 medium fresh fruit = tennis ball

1 cup of raw vegetables = light bulb

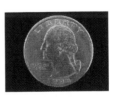

1 teaspoon of oil = 25c in diameter

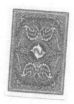

3 ounces of meat = deck of cards

Some notes on serving sizes of foods that we are commonly served.

You are normally served about 40 chips in a bowl (tortilla chips) when 10-12 is a serving – 4 x larger than you need to eat and an additional 300 calories.

You are normally served a 24 ounce regular soda, and 1 serving is about 12 ounces. Adding 150 more calories to your beverage.

You are normally served a 4 ounce bagel, plain and a 1.5 ounce plain bagel is the appropriate serving size, so you get about 200 calories more than you need.

At the cash register in your favorite cafeteria, they have chocolate chip cookies wrapped in cellophane. The usual size of the cookie is 5 ounces, 700 calories, and 20 grams of fat – but a normal serving of a cookie is about 1 ounce and 140 calories, with 4 grams of fat. The difference is about 550 calories!

Watch out for terms like: combo, ultimate, Jumbo, Deluxe, Value Meal, Super size – all of those indicate that you are getting a meal that is much bigger than the normal serving size. And at a fast food restaurant, you can bet you don't get whole grain, whole wheat buns and plenty of vegetables.

GETTING STARTED NOW

You may have been told to watch all kinds of nutrients as part of a kidney diet. Truth be told, very few matter until you get the basics in place with your meal planning. You have taken a great big step in the right direction by reading this book.

You should get your general diet in order and on the right track so you are positioned to make the other changes that might be necessary to slow the progression of your kidney failure. It's easier to make changes incrementally, so start with the changes in this book to have a good beginning.

NEXT STEPS

1. Start with controlling the nutrients we discussed – protein, carbohydrate and fat. Count your calories and understand what you are eating. I encourage you to write down all that you eat and quantify it for at least 3 days.

2. You will understand where you need to make changes much easier if you have made the effort to write down your meals, and indentify your problem areas.

3. Write out your meals for the next week. Cook the dinners that you like and compose a plan for your daily meals – lunches, snacks, breakfast and supper. It's easier once you have done one using the information in this book.

4. Reduce your use of high potassium and high phosphorus foods so you can feel comfortable choosing from the foods on the list and being on your right diet. You will start to feel better in days, not weeks, once you are eating better and not experiencing the signs of uremia and other toxic substances in your blood. Make note of the changes you experience and discuss questions about your labs or items specific to your health with your physician.

5. Send me an email with any questions about this book to contact@renaldiethq.com

If you would like to know when we have new books coming out – please go to:

http://www.renaldiethq.com/go/booknotify/book1

Sign up for the email list and we will let you know when the next book is released in the series.

Made in the USA
Lexington, KY
02 May 2014